Boiled Egg Diet

Eat Smart for Quick Results & Discover How to Keep the Weight Off

Thomas Rohmer

Copyright © 2018

Disclaimer:

This guide has been created for informational and reference
purposes only. The author, publisher, and any other
affiliated parties cannot be held in any way accountable for
any personal injuries or damage allegedly resulting from the
information contained herein, or from any misuse of such
guidance. Although strict measures have been taken to
provide accurate information, the parties involved with the
creation and publication of this guide take no responsibility
for any issues that many arise from alleged discrepancies
contained herein. It is strongly recommended that you
consult a physician, personal trainer, and nutritionist prior
to commencing this or any other workout or diet plan. This
guide is not a substitute for professional personal guidance
from a qualified medical professional. If you feel pain or
discomfort at any point during exercises contained herein,
cease the activity immediately and seek medical guidance.

Before You Begin:

Get the Latest Scoop on the Most Cutting Edge Info on Health & Fitness!

As thanks for picking up this book, I'd love to offer you the chance to maximize your results by getting exclusive info on health and fitness.

You'll be the first to know when I publish new books, and you'll receive exclusive content on health and fitness that I only share with people on my list.

Simply visit the link directly below and get started on the path to the healthiest version of yourself today!

https://rohmerfitness.lpages.co/kindle-sign-up/

Table Of Contents

Introduction:

Losing weight is hard. Each and every year, millions of Americans go on a diet to try and lose weight and very few are actually successful.

Not only that, but even fewer are able to actually keep the weight off. What are you supposed to do? It can feel rather hopeless.

Most diets set you up to fail from the get-go. They force you to eat boring foods all of the time, or they don't give you fast results.

This makes you worry and doubt that what you're doing is worth the effort. Fortunately, the boiled egg diet is the solution that can help you not only lose weight but keep it off for good.

Additionally, the boiled egg diet will help you lose weight quickly, which will help you stay motivated and want to continue moving forward. The thing is though, you have to be smart with the way in which you approach the boiled egg diet.

The reason is that the boiled egg diet only lasts for two weeks. What are you supposed to do after that initial two-week period is over?

This is where most diet plans will leave you in the dust, and this is why rebound weight gain occurs. I don't want this to happen to you.

That's why I've dedicated an entire chapter to how to smoothly transition out of the boiled egg diet once it's over.

Not only that, but I'm also going to share with you when the best time is for you to start another boiled egg diet if you want to lose more weight. With this approach, fat loss will be inevitable—let's dive in and get started...

Chapter 1: What is the Boiled Egg Diet?

The boiled egg diet is a weight loss diet that can help you lose up to 24 pounds in as little as two weeks. Of course, you may not lose 24 pounds over two weeks, but you'll still lose a good amount of weight in a short period of time.

Not only that, but two weeks are manageable and a short enough timeframe to help keep you motivated. With most typical diets, you have no timetable for what type of results you can expect.

That can be really discouraging, which is honestly why I think most people give up on their diet plan. It's not because people are lazy, it has more to do with the fact that most diets aren't that good, and they set you up to fail from the get-go.

Most diet and weight loss plans only care about making a sale, and they don't care about your long-term success. That's why I really want to show you how to approach the boiled egg diet in a way that'll set you up for success.

And as you can probably guess, the core of the diet centers around eating boiled eggs. However, that's not the only thing that you'll be consuming.

You'll also eat various fruits, vegetables, and lean meats among other things. I'll cover more of the specific meal plan in a later chapter, but for now you need to know that you'll primarily be eating healthy foods while on this diet plan.

The reason for this is because what you eat does matter greatly. Clean foods such as fruits and vegetables are high in fiber, which will help to keep you fuller for a longer period of time.

On the other hand, if you eat primarily junk food to eat alongside your boiled eggs, then you'll spike your blood sugar and have random cravings throughout the day. That's not something you want to be battling with all day when your calories are being restricted!

That's why you must have a balance between eating healthy foods, but still allow yourself to enjoy some of your favorite foods from time to time. Seriously who do you know that's gone on a diet where they eat nothing but healthy foods and was able to stick with it for a long time?

I sure don't know of anyone! If you only try to eat healthy foods, you'll eventually go insane.

That's why when the initial two week period of the boiled egg diet is over, you'll eat in a way that'll help give you a bit of a break from the intense dieting you were doing during the previous two weeks.

It all comes down to balance in the end. Eating too much junk food is bad because junk food generally contains more calories and it'll lead to weight gain.

On the flip side, eating nothing but clean foods will make you want to quit. And don't worry, in later chapters I'll show you how to strike that balance.

This is meant to give you a general understanding of what to do during and after the boiled egg diet. Now it's time to get into some more specifics, let's start with how your body works in regards to weight loss...

Chapter 2: How the Boiled Egg Diet Works

When you think of a diet, what do you typically think of? You probably think of something like eating nothing but wholesome foods in an effort to lose weight.

The thing is though; do you have to eat healthy in order to lose weight? The answer to that is no.

In fact, the only thing you need in order to lose weight is a caloric deficit. A caloric deficit is when you burn off more calories than you consume.

So for example, if you burn off 2,000 calories a day, then you would need to eat less than 2,000 calories a day in order to start losing weight. On the other hand, when you eat more calories than you burn off, you're in a caloric surplus.

This is how you gain weight. Unfortunately, most people have no clue what a caloric deficit or a caloric surplus is.

This is really sad because this is the basis for how your body gains/loses weight. You could theoretically eat nothing but healthy foods, but if you overeat those foods and still end up in a surplus, then you won't be losing any weight.

Therefore, it's important to understand how many calories you're burning off in a day, so you can ensure that you're eating under that amount for weight loss.

If You Want Something to Blame, Blame Biology

Everyday your body needs energy to perform daily functions such as breathing, digesting food, and organ function among other things. Where does your body get this energy from in order to carry out these tasks?

It gets it from the foods that you eat. Food contains calories. Calories are essentially a measurement of the amount of energy a certain food item contains.

Therefore the more calories something contains, the more energy you're giving your body to use to carry out its daily functions and any other activities you might be doing such as exercise. Of course, if you eat too many calories, you're body will store the leftovers that it didn't need as fat for later use.

This might seem like a big let down, but we probably wouldn't be here today if it weren't for our bodies acting in this manner. Back in the days of our ancestors, food was scarce.

You didn't know where your next meal was going to come from. That's why when you did find food, it was usually when you would hunt down a big animal such as a buffalo.

Then you would get to feast for the next couple of days. Your body will then store the remaining calories as fat because it would be awhile before you found a significant amount of food again.

This is also why we are so compelled to eat sugary and salty foods. These foods are higher in calories, so our ancestors would need to seek out and eat as much of these foods as they could when they found them.

Obviously when you fast forward to the present day, this biological programming hurts us more than it helps us. It's easier and more convenient to get food now more than ever.

You can get in your car at any time and drive through a fast food restaurant. Heck if you want to be even lazier, you can have food delivered to your house.

Sugary and salty foods are easy to find as well. It doesn't help that companies want to expose us to these foods to help make a profit at the cost of our health. Back in the day, when food was scarcer, this benefited us.

Now days, it seems to hurt us more than it helps us. That's why you have to be smart in how you approach burning fat.

Treating it like a sprint where you eat extremely low amounts of calories for a long period of time is only going to cause you to crash and burn. Instead be smart and work with your biology.

Eat in a pattern like your ancestors would. Your ancestors would have periods of time where they would consume lower amounts of calories, and then they would have periods of time where they would consume higher amounts of calories.

This is exactly what we're going to mimic with the boiled egg diet. While you're following the boiled egg diet, your calories are going to be restricted.

This is going to be like someone back in the day eating low amounts of calories from foods that they could gather while they waited for the next big hunt. Then you're going to balance this with periods where you'll be eating a higher amount of calories.

Of course, it won't be too high to where you end up gaining a bunch of weight. And this is going to mimic our ancestors finding a big animal to feast on for a while. When you approach things in this strategic manner, you're way more likely to achieve fat loss success.

How Many Calories Do You Burn Off Per Day?

As I just mentioned, every day your body needs energy in order to carry out its daily functions. Your body gets this energy from the foods that you eat.

The total amount of calories that you burn off in a given day is known as your resting metabolic rate. And it's actually quite simple to determine your resting metabolic rate.

All you need to do is take your current bodyweight and multiply it by 13. I'll use myself as an example:

Current bodyweight= 207 pounds

Resting metabolic rate: 207 x13=2,691

Knowing that I burn off 2,691 calories every day, this would mean that:

- If I eat less than 2,691 calories per day, then I would be in a caloric deficit, and I'd start to lose weight.
- If I eat more than 2,691 calories per day, then I would be in a caloric surplus, and I'd start to gain weight.
- If I eat right at 2,691 calories per day, then I would be at maintenance, and I would neither gain nor lose weight.

Simply knowing your resting metabolic rate isn't enough. The reason for this is because if I eat around 2,691 calories per day, then that still won't be enough for me to lose weight.

So the real question is, how many calories below 2,691 should I eat in order to lose weight? For example, I could eat 2,600 calories and create a daily caloric deficit of 91 calories, but that would have me losing weight at an extremely slow pace.

That's why it's important to lose weight at a rate that'll keep you encouraged, but not so low that you're not able to maintain it. Later on, I'll share with you the exact amounts you should eat at when you're not following the boiled egg diet.

When you are following the boiled egg diet however, you won't have to worry about the size of the caloric deficit you're creating. The reason for this is because you'll simply eat as the meal plan tells you to and forget about the rest.

When you're following the meal plan of the boiled egg diet, you'll be eating a low enough amount of calories that you'll be in a large caloric deficit. I mean you can lose up to 24 pounds in as little as two weeks for crying out loud!

What Makes the Boiled Egg Diet so Special?

Right now you might be thinking, "So then what is it that makes the boiled egg diet so special? Can't I eat how I like, and as long as I'm in a caloric deficit, I'll be good to go?"

The answer to that is yes, you could do that and get results, however you're much better off following the boiled egg diet. There are multiple reasons for this:

1. The boiled egg diet will give you a structured plan.
2. It's extremely easy to follow and doesn't involve a lot of time to prepare and eat the foods.
3. It allows you to mimic an eating pattern that's similar to the way in which our ancient ancestors ate.

Of course, when it comes to the boiled egg diet, there isn't anything too particularly special about the foods that you'll be eating. The main goal with the boiled egg diet is the same as any other diet out there—get you in a caloric deficit for a prolonged period of time.

However, the boiled egg diet will provide you with the benefits that I just mentioned, which are critical. They are the difference between frustration and no results and success.

Chapter 3: Boiled Egg Diet Meal Plan

Ok now it's time to get into the fun part. We're going to go over exactly what you're going to be eating during the two weeks that you're on the boiled egg diet.

During this two week boiled egg diet, you won't have to worry too much about tracking and measuring your calories (more on how to do this later). The reason for this is because the meal plan will take care of all of that for you.

You'll be eating a low enough amount of calories during these two weeks to be in a pretty big caloric deficit, so you could simply eat what it tells you to and forget about the rest. However, once this initial two-week period is up, you'll definitely want to make sure that you're keeping track of your caloric intake.

Most people overestimate the amount of calories that they eat. This is definitely something that you'll want to avoid because it means that you won't be getting any results.

Once you start to track and measure things, you might be surprised to realize how many calories it was that you were eating. I'll share with you in exact detail what to do after this initial two-week period, but for now your main focus is the boiled egg diet. Here's the boiled egg diet meal plan:

Day 1 Monday:

Breakfast:

Two boiled eggs
One piece of citrus fruit of your choosing

Lunch:

2 sweet potatoes and 1 piece of fruit of your choosing

Dinner:

Large Chicken salad

Day 2 Tuesday:

Breakfast:

Two boiled eggs and 1 piece of citrus fruit

Lunch:

Medium Chicken salad

Dinner:

Two eggs (cooked how you like), your choice of vegetables, and 1 piece of fruit

Day 3 Wednesday:

Breakfast:

Two boiled eggs and 1 piece of citrus fruit

Lunch:

Medium or Large chicken salad

Dinner:

One tomato, 1 slice of low-fat cheese, and one slice of whole-wheat bread

Day 4 Thursday:

Breakfast:

Two boiled eggs and 1 piece of citrus fruit

Lunch:

2 eggs (cooked how you like), 1 slice of low-fat cheese, and vegetables of your choosing

Dinner:

Large chicken salad

Day 5 Friday:

Breakfast:

Two boiled eggs and 1 piece of citrus fruit

Lunch:

Vegetables of your choosing and two eggs cooked how you like

Dinner:

Large tuna salad or another type of fish of your choosing

Day 6 Saturday:

Breakfast:

Two boiled eggs and 1 piece of citrus fruit

Lunch:

Your choice of fruit

Dinner:

Large chicken salad

Day 7 Sunday:

Breakfast:

Two boiled eggs and 1 piece of citrus fruit

Lunch:

Chicken with a tomato and your choice of cooked vegetables

Day 8 Monday:

Breakfast:

Two boiled eggs and 1 piece of citrus fruit

Lunch:

Medium chicken salad

Dinner:

Two eggs cooked how you like, one piece of citrus fruit, and a vegetable salad

Day 9 Tuesday:

Breakfast:

Two boiled eggs and 1 piece of citrus fruit

Lunch:

Two eggs cooked how you like and your choice of cooked vegetables

Dinner:

Your choice of a fish salad

Day 10 Wednesday:

Breakfast:

Two boiled eggs and 1 piece of citrus fruit

Lunch:

Medium chicken salad

Dinner:

Two eggs cooked how you like, 1 orange, and a vegetable salad

Day 11 Thursday:

Breakfast:

Two boiled eggs and 1 piece of citrus fruit

Lunch:

1 slice of low-fat cheese, two eggs cooked how you like, and cooked vegetables

Dinner:

Large chicken salad

Day 12 Friday:

Breakfast:

Two boiled eggs and 1 piece of citrus fruit

Lunch:

Medium fish salad

Dinner:

Two eggs cooked how you like and a vegetable salad

Day 13 Saturday:

Breakfast:

Two boiled eggs and 1 piece of citrus fruit

Lunch:

Medium chicken salad

Dinner:

Your choice of fruit

Day 14 Sunday:

Breakfast:

Two boiled eggs and 1 piece of citrus fruit

Lunch:

Chicken and cooked vegetables

Dinner:

Same as lunch—chicken and cooked vegetables

You'll notice that there's not any mention of portion sizes listed. Sometimes you might be eating a medium chicken salad and other times a large chicken salad.

Don't get too caught up in the portion sizes. Eat a healthy amount when it comes to the fruits, vegetables, and sizes of your salads.

Eat enough to where you feel satisfied, but not stuffed. You'll also notice that for some of the meals you'll only be eating fruit. In this case, eat enough to where you feel satisfied.

It doesn't have to be a specific number of pieces that you eat. All of the foods that you're going to be consuming on the boiled egg diet are healthy, so it's going to be hard to overeat them.

Therefore don't get so caught up in the specifics of how much of a certain food to eat. For example, breakfast is always the same with two boiled eggs and a piece of citrus fruit.

However, if one morning you're feeling particularly hungry go ahead and eat another piece or two of fruit if you have to. It won't ruin the diet by any means.

Chapter 4: How to Prevent the Vicious Yo-Yo Dieting Cycle

There's nothing worse than to lose a bunch of weight only to gain it all back in a few months. The real key to success with weight loss really isn't about losing the weight; it's about making sure that it stays off for good.

Sadly this is something that most people struggle with. It's not hard for someone to push himself hard and lose a good chunk of weight, however the real challenge comes in afterwards.

What are you going to do in order to keep the weight off? Most dieters never really consider this.

Unfortunately most diets out there are set up in a way to have you lose weight quickly (which isn't a bad thing necessarily), but they leave you clueless for what to do once the diet ends. Many diets are too severe to continue doing for long periods of time, therefore it would be extremely challenging to continue following it for any significant length of time.

This is why most people who want to lose weight fall into the vicious cycle of yo-yo dieting. Yo-yo dieting is where you go on an extreme diet to lose weight quickly.

Then once the diet is over, you go back to your normal eating patterns. This then causes you to gain all of the weight back that you worked so hard to lose in the first place.

Then once you're unsatisfied with how you look, you repeat the cycle by going on another diet to lose weight only to gain it all back once the diet ends. That's why if you want to be successful, you must have a serious plan of action for what you'll do once the diet is over.

Hardly anybody does, and that's why so many people gain back all of the weight that they lost. Now I'm going to be straight with you, the boiled egg diet is on the extreme side when it comes to diets.

It only lasts for two weeks, which is a good thing because I don't think most people could handle it for much longer than that. You definitely wouldn't be able to keep up with something like this for years and years to come.

Therefore, you must be smart with what you do once the initial two-week period is up, and that's what this chapter is going to help you do.

How to Transition Out of the Boiled Egg Diet

Ok so once you finish the boiled egg diet is that it? Do you go back to your normal eating habits and forget about everything else?

No definitely not! That's a great way to erase any weight loss that did occur during the boiled egg diet.

Instead what you're going to have to focus on now is how many calories you're eating. Yes this means that you're going to have to track and measure how many calories it is that you're eating on a daily basis.

If you don't, then you're simply guessing and that will lead to sloppy results. On the boiled egg diet, you don't have to worry about tracking your calories because you're going to be in a significant caloric deficit by following the meal plan.

However, now you're going to want to recall your resting metabolic rate that we calculated earlier by multiplying your bodyweight by 13. This is the total number of calories you burn off in a given day.

Of course, though, you're not going to initially eat right at maintenance. Chances are that you probably still want to lose more weight than you initially did with the boiled egg diet.

That's why during parts of this transition phase, you're still going to be eating in a caloric deficit, it just won't be as large of a caloric deficit. During the boiled egg diet, you're going to be consuming around 1,100-1,400 calories per day.

And let's say for example that your resting metabolic rate is 2,200 calories. This means that you were in a pretty big caloric deficit while you were on the boiled egg diet.

After the boiled egg diet is over, you don't want to immediately jump into eating 2,200 calories per day. You won't continue losing any weight that way.

Instead, you're better off eating more calories than you were on the boiled egg diet but still less than maintenance. Here's a breakdown of how I would transition out of the boiled egg diet:

My resting metabolic rate is 2,691

Weeks 1 and 2: follow the boiled egg diet, total calories per day—approximately 1,100-1,400

Week 3: eat at a caloric deficit of 500 calories per day. This would have me eating roughly 2,191 calories per day.

Week 4: eat at a caloric deficit of 250 calories per day. In my case, I would eat 2,441 calories per day.

Weeks 5 and 6: eat at a caloric deficit of 100 calories per day. In my case, I would eat 2,591 calories per day.

Weeks 7 and 8: eat at maintenance calories. In my case, I would eat 2,691 calories per day.

To put things into perspective better, eating at a caloric deficit of 500 calories per day will have you losing roughly one pound per week (1). Then when you're in a caloric deficit of 250 calories per day, you'll be losing about .5 pound per week.

Now you might be wondering why it is that the transition period is drawn out for such a long time. The reason is because you did a heavy amount of dieting during the two-week period of the boiled egg diet.

After that's over, you want to ease off the gas pedal and give yourself some time to recuperate. The majority of your weight loss will occur during the two-week period of the boiled egg diet.

The rest of the time after that isn't about losing weight as much as it's about recovering and preparing yourself for the next boiled egg diet. Yes in an ideal world, you'd be able to go non-stop with the boiled egg diet until you reach your ideal weight.

However, that approach won't work. You'll run yourself into the ground and quit before you reach your goal bodyweight. That's why you have to alternate between periods of going hard and periods of taking it easy.

Imagine it like a sprint. Ideally, you'd be able to sprint at maximum speed for miles on end without tiring.

The thing is though, you can't run at max speeds for a long period of time. That's why the best thing you can do is sprint for as long as you can.

Then once you get tired, you take a break and allow yourself time to recuperate. Then once you have your energy back, you can go back to sprinting at max speed.

This is similar to how things will be approached with the boiled egg diet. Picture the boiled egg diet like a sprint.

During this timeframe, you'll go all out and lose a bunch of weight. By the end of it, you'll be worn out and need to take a break from the heavy dieting.

This is where the transition phase comes into play. It'll be like taking a break from the sprint, allowing you to fully recover.

Then once you're feeling good again, you can go at it again with another boiled egg diet and continue to repeat the process until you hit your goal.

How to Vary the Transition Period Based on Your Needs

The cool thing is that you don't have to follow the transition period exactly as I laid it out if you don't want to. You might find that you do better on a shorter timeframe or even a longer one.

If that's the case for you, then certainly don't hesitate to make the change. Here are a few examples of how you could shorten or lengthen the transition period to better suit your needs:

- Weeks 1 and 2: boiled egg diet consuming around 1,100-1,400 calories per day
- Week 3: eat at a caloric deficit of 500 calories.
- Week 4: eat at a caloric deficit of 250 calories.
- Week 5: eat at maintenance.

- Weeks 6 and 7: boiled egg diet

Or:

- Weeks 1 and 2: boiled egg diet
- Weeks 3 and 4: eat at a caloric deficit of 500 calories.
- Weeks 5 and 6: eat at a caloric deficit of 250 calories.
- Weeks 7 and 8: eat at a caloric deficit of 100 calories.
- Weeks 9 and 10: eat at maintenance.
- Weeks 11 and 12: boiled egg diet

If you wanted to, you could even change things up to where you follow the boiled egg diet for only one week instead of two. You could then test out different transition periods and see how you feel. For example:

- Week 1: boiled egg diet
- Week 2: eat at a caloric deficit of 500 calories
- Week 3: eat at a caloric deficit of 250 calories
- Week 4: eat at a caloric deficit of 100 calories
- Week 5: eat at maintenance
- Week 6: boiled egg diet

Or:

- Week 1: boiled egg diet
- Weeks 2 and 3: eat at a caloric deficit of 500 calories
- Weeks 4 and 5: eat at a caloric deficit of 250 calories
- Weeks 6 and 7: eat at a caloric deficit of 100 calories
- Weeks 8 and 9: eat at maintenance
- Week 10: boiled egg diet

Note: you can also change the size of your caloric deficits during the transition phase as well. For example, if you'd rather eat in a smaller deficit of let's say 300 calories instead of 500 you can certainly do so.

You're also free to create a larger deficit than 500 calories as well if you want to. After going through this process and getting some experience with it, you'll get a better feel for how large of a deficit you can handle.

It's all about experimenting and seeing what works best for you. Everyone is unique and different so what works for someone else may not work perfectly for you. I'd recommend starting out with the first transition plan that I laid out, but afterwards, tweak it to suit your needs.

What Should You Eat During the Transition Phase?

When you're following the boiled egg diet, what you're going to eat is pretty simple—just eat what the plan tells you to. However, figuring out what to eat during the weeks when you're not following the boiled egg diet can be a bit more challenging.

It's better for me to tell you the basic outlines and principles of how you should eat rather than for me to try and tell you what to eat all of the time. By understanding the basic principles of fat loss, and the key differences between macronutrient quality, you'll be much more adaptable and prepared for success.

The reason for this is because you won't always be able to follow a meal plan exactly as it's laid out. Sure when it's only for a short timeframe such as two-weeks with the boiled egg diet, that's not so bad and it can easily be done.

But doing that for the majority of your life would be hard to follow. Imagine you go to a party or some other social event. Chances are good that you're probably not going to be "that guy" who brings his own food to the event.

And if that's the case, then you're going to be forced to eat whatever food is available to you. If all you know how to do is follow a meal plan, then you'll freeze up.

You won't know what you should and shouldn't eat. You'll likely make up an excuse like, "It's only one night, this can't mess up my results too badly!"

When the reality is that it certainly can make you take a step backwards. If on the other hand, you knew how to adapt yourself to the situation, you'd be much better off.

You'd know for example, that you burn off 2,200 calories a day for instance and that you usually eat a 750-calorie dinner. Since this is a special event that doesn't happen all of the time, you know that you'll likely want to eat more than 750 calories for dinner.

Therefore, you could eat a smaller breakfast and lunch and save those extra calories for the event. This way you'll still be able to enjoy yourself, but you won't have to worry about gaining weight.

That's why you need to focus more on these guidelines that I'm going to outline for you instead of worrying so much about what specific foods you should be eating. Remember the main thing that matters for weight loss is creating a caloric deficit!

That needs to be the number one priority for you to consider and what you eat is secondary.

Guideline #1: Understand the importance of calorie quality

Is a calorie a calorie? Is 200 calories of potato chips the same as 200 calories of fruits and vegetables? Well yes and no.

The overall amount of calories is the same. So in terms of creating a caloric deficit, it would be the same.

Trying to say that 200 calories of this food isn't equal to 200 calories of that food is like saying a yard of wood isn't the same length as a yard of metal. The length is the same, however the materials that they're made of is different.

The same goes for calories. The total number of calories from the example is the same.

However, the quality of those calories are very different much like wood is very different from metal. The potato chips are empty calories, meaning that they won't provide you with very much nutritional value for how many calories they're providing you with.

Due to this lack of nutrition, the potato chips won't do a good job of keeping you full for a long period of time. They'll also make you feel low on energy, and you'll likely have to consume more calories in order to get full.

On the other hand, the fruits and vegetables contain lots of vitamins, minerals, and fiber. This is going to help keep you fuller for a longer period of time.

Many people falsely believe that if they eat healthy foods they're guaranteed to lose weight. This certainly isn't the case because it's still possible to overeat healthy foods.

You can eat foods like oatmeal and avocados and be in a caloric surplus. On the flip side, you can eat junk food like candy and pastries and still be in a caloric deficit.

Sure it's not a sustainable way to maintain a caloric deficit, but the point is to show you that you don't necessarily gain weight by eating junk nor lose weight by eating healthy.

Ultimately though, eating healthy the majority of the time is key when you're calories are being restricted in order to lose weight. If you waste all of your allotted calories for the day on junk food, then you're likely going to feel hungry all day or crash and overeat.

With this being said, should you eat nothing but healthy foods all of the time? The answer to that is definitely not!

I'll share with you in another guideline how to strike a good balance between eating junk food and eating clean foods. Eating your favorite treats from time to time is a good thing.

If you only ate clean foods your whole life, you'd go insane. Eating junk food will help you to keep your sanity and allow you to follow a sustainable diet approach. Like I said though, the key to this is finding a balance.

Guideline #2: Follow the 85% Golden Rule

Ok so you know you shouldn't eat healthy 100% of the time, but you also know that eating junk food all of the time isn't a good idea either. What should you do then?

You need to follow my golden rule which states that you should eat clean and healthy foods roughly 85% of the time. The other 15% of the time, you can eat how you please.

And of course, you can distribute the 15% however it is that you like. You could do something like enjoying a small bag of potato chips every day, eat any meal that you like every 2-3 days, or even save up for one day of the week where you eat however you like.

Of course, you'll want to make sure that you don't overeat and you're still eating the correct amount of total calories. And you don't have to worry about it being exactly 15% either.

Sometimes it might be lower than 15%, other times it might be higher than 15%. The main point is to focus on being in the realm of 15% and to realize that as long as you're eating healthy the majority of the time you should be good to go.

In terms of what you should be eating for healthy foods, I would focus on eating foods like fruits, vegetables, lean meats, sweet potatoes, brown rice, oatmeal, nuts, and avocados among other things.

Basically, try to think about how our ancestors would've eaten back in the hunter and gather days. If they wouldn't have been able to eat it, then it probably isn't a wholesome food and should be counted towards your 15% junk food.

Guideline #3: Distribute your calories out however you like

Most people eat a standard breakfast, lunch, and dinner, but most people feel like the number of calories you eat at each meal has to be the same. You don't have to eat the same number of calories for each meal, you can distribute out your calories however it is that you like.

Do what works best for you. Maybe you like to eat bigger dinners and smaller breakfasts.

If this is the case for you, and you're eating a total of 2,200 calories per day for example, then you could eat 500 calories for breakfast, 700 calories for lunch, and then 1,000 calories for dinner. Break it up however you like and do what works best for your schedule.

Guideline #4: Eat as frequently or infrequently as you like

Many people believe that it's better to eat smaller meals more frequently throughout the day because this will boost

your metabolism. The research actually shows that meal
frequency doesn't matter for weight loss (2).

For example, eating 6 meals per day is the same as eating 1
meal per day as long as the total number of calories is the
same in both cases. Therefore, eat as frequently or
infrequently as you like.

Do what works best for you and your schedule. For example,
if you're not hungry in the morning, then don't feel obligated
to eat breakfast. Instead, save those calories for later on in
the day when you actually want to eat them.

If you follow these guidelines, then you'll be much better off
during your transition period when you're not following the
boiled egg diet as compared to someone who only knows how
to follow a meal plan.

How to Track and Measure Your Caloric Intake

The last thing we need to talk about before we wrap up this
chapter is how you should track and measure your calories.
All of these guidelines and formulas are great, but they don't
mean anything if you don't know how to measure the
amount of calories that you're eating.

The first thing you need to do is go to the app store and
download a calorie counting app. Typing in something like
macro calculator or calorie counting app should work fine.

Some of them will be paid and others free. Don't hesitate to
pay a couple of dollars to get a good app. It'll pay for itself
multiple times over.

Most of the apps have really cool features where you can use
your phone to scan the barcode of a food label and it'll
instantly track the info for you. You can also type in the food

item that you're eating and it'll pop up with the info and then log it for you.

This makes it really simple, which is key. If something is a pain to do, then you're probably not going to stick with it.

On the other hand, you could go old school and keep track of your calories with a pen and paper. This is going to be quite a bit harder to do, but it can still be done.

You'll simply look up the nutrition information of the foods you're eating online and then record it on paper. All you have to worry about is the total amount of calories that you're eating.

And as long as you're following the rule of eating healthy 85% of the time, you'll be good to go. The other thing you'll want to get is a food scale.

You can usually get one of these for around $10 and this is going to help you measure the amount of food that you're eating. The apps work great, but you have to know the amount of the food that you're eating, otherwise you're simply taking your best guess.

For example, if you're eating 20 grams of chicken, you can look up how many calories are in 20 grams of chicken, but you first have to know that you're consuming 20 grams of chicken. The only way you would know this for sure is if you have a food scale.

So now you might be thinking, what am I supposed to do when I'm away from home and I'm not able to use a food scale or track my calories? A lot of restaurants will have their nutrition information either online or on the menu, which makes it easy to track because the calories have already been counted for you.

If you're eating at a place that doesn't have the nutrition info readily available, then you'll have to take your best guess. Over time you'll get better at this, but at first you might not be too accurate with it.

It's a good rule of thumb to overestimate the amount of calories that you're eating to be on the safe side. Most people underestimate the amount of calories that they're eating and it only ends up hurting them when they don't get the results that they want.

It's better to overestimate the amount of calories in the foods that you're eating so that way you can still be on track to hit your weight loss goal. That's really all there is to it.

Yes counting calories can be a pain in the neck at times, but it's something you have to do because what gets measured gets managed. If you're not willing to measure your calories during the transition phase, then you may or may not end up with the results that you want.

Chapter 5: What to Do When You Reach Your Goal Bodyweight

Let's say you've followed the outline from the last chapter and you hit your goal bodyweight. What should you do now?

Do you keep on following the boiled egg diet? Do you eat however you want? In this chapter, I'm going to share with you what changes and what doesn't once you hit your target bodyweight.

How Will You Know What Your Goal Bodyweight Is?

Right now you might be wondering what your goal bodyweight is. Unfortunately, there's no formula to say that a male or female who is this tall should weigh this much.

Yes there's something called body mass index or BMI, but this is simply a height to weight ratio. It doesn't measure how much muscle or fat is on your body.

Take myself for example. I'm 6'4" and I weigh 207 pounds. This means that my BMI is 25.2.

According to the BMI chart having a BMI of over 25 means that you're overweight, and having a BMI of over 30 means that you're obese. Like I said earlier, the BMI chart doesn't take into account muscle mass.

I wouldn't consider myself an overweight individual by any means, but according to the BMI chart I'm overweight. Most professional athletes would be in the overweight or obese category as well even though they're some of the fittest people in the world.

So if something like BMI isn't reliable, then what is? What can you use to determine what your goal bodyweight should be?

The answer to that is you won't know until you get there. Once you like the way that you look, step on the scale and see how much you weigh—that's your goal bodyweight.

Of course this would mean that you wouldn't know exactly how much you need to weigh as you're trying to lose weight. That's completely ok!

Instead you can simply take your best guess as to what your goal bodyweight is and you can adjust as you need to along the way. For example, let's say someone weighs 200 pounds, and he knows he needs to lose weight, but he's not sure how much.

He could take a guess and say that his goal bodyweight is 165 pounds. Then once he gets down to 180 pounds, let's pretend he's pretty happy with the progress that he's made and he knows that he's close to where he wants to end up.

He could readjust his goal bodyweight to 175 pounds for example. Then once he gets down to 175 pounds, he can see how he looks and if he's satisfied or not.

If so, then great! If not, then he'll need to lower his target bodyweight again down to 170 and see how he looks at that bodyweight.

Even though you'll have to take your best guess as to what your goal bodyweight is, it's still a good idea to pick a goal bodyweight because it gives you something to aim for. Ultimately the mirror is the best judge.

If you're happy with how you look in the mirror, then you're good to go. A number on the scale is arbitrary and it doesn't have much meaning.

How you look on the other hand does matter, that's why you want to lose weight in the first place. You want to lose weight so you'll look better, get healthier, and have more energy.

You're not interested in losing weight so a number on the scale will be lower. Seriously a weight scale is a machine, you don't need to worry about impressing it!

How Often Should You Weigh Yourself?

The next thing you might be wondering is how often you should weigh yourself, or if you should even weigh yourself at all! Yes you still need to weigh yourself because the scale will help you know if you're heading in the right direction or not.

It's similar to the reason why you measure and count your calories—if you don't measure it, then you have no idea where you're going! The thing is though, you can certainly go overboard when it comes to weighing yourself, and this can cause you to second guess yourself and doubt if what you're doing is working.

For example, if you weigh yourself everyday, then you might weigh 170 pounds one day and 172 the next day. What gives?

Did you actually gain 2 pounds in one day? The answer to that is no, you didn't gain 2 pounds in one day.

What's actually going on is that your bodyweight is fluctuating. In fact, your body weight can fluctuate by up to as much as five pounds.

Your bodyweight can fluctuate depending on if you just ate a meal, how hydrated you are, etc. That's also why the time of day when you weigh yourself matters as well.

If you weigh yourself first thing in the morning do you think you're going to weigh the same as if you weigh yourself in the evening after eating three meals? No way!

So then what is the best way to go about weighing yourself? You should only weigh yourself once per week.

This will help to account for any fluctuations in body weight and help you determine if you've actually lost or gained weight. It'll also keep you from going crazy because you won't have to worry about your bodyweight going up and down all of the time.

For example, if you step on the scale on Monday and weigh 170 pounds, and then the following Monday you weigh yourself again and weigh 168 pounds, you can be sure that you've actually lost 2 pounds. Whereas if you weigh yourself every day and the scale says you "lost" two pounds, it could simply be a fluctuation in your bodyweight and not actual weight loss.

The next thing you'll want to do is weigh yourself at the same time. The best way to make this consistent is to weigh yourself first thing in the morning right after you go to the bathroom.

This way you won't have any food in your stomach, and your hydration levels should be roughly the same as well. Measuring your bodyweight at any other time of the day will lead to inconsistencies.

If you follow those two guidelines, then you'll be good to go. Of course, there will be some weeks where you might not lose any weight or lose as much weight as you wanted to for the week.

When this happens don't freak out. You can always pick yourself back up and have a better upcoming week.

Think about it like a stock. Does a stock of a company always go up and up and up, but never down? Of course not!

Stocks fluctuate up and down all of the time! I'm not saying that your bodyweight should be going up and down like a stock, but don't expect for things to be smooth sailing all of the time because that won't happen.

Some weeks you might gain a little bit of weight, other weeks you won't lose weight, and some weeks you'll lose more than you expected. The key is to not get too upset when things don't go your way.

This is a long-term game you're playing here. It's not won or lost over the course of one week.

Stay focused, and keep your eyes on the prize. If you're able to do that, then you'll be able to bounce back the following week. On the other hand, if you get frustrated and upset, then you'll likely quit out of despair sooner than later.

How Things Change When You Reach Your Target Bodyweight

This is something interesting that most people don't think about—what are you supposed to do once you hit your target bodyweight? Most people who go on a diet never reach this point sadly, so it's not something people usually consider.

The truth is that not much will change from what you were doing to lose weight than what you will do to maintain your weight. When you're trying to lose weight, you eat in a caloric deficit.

Now that you want to maintain your weight, you're not going to continue eating in a caloric deficit. If you did that, then you would continue to lose weight, and that's not what you want anymore.

Instead, you'll want to eat enough calories to where you don't gain or lose weight. This is tricky because most people will go back to eating the way they did before they started their weight loss diet.

If you do that, then you'll likely put yourself back into a caloric surplus and slowly start to gain back all of the weight that you lost. You might think that you can go back to your normal eating habits and be okay, but this is wishful thinking.

Don't deceive yourself into thinking that you can eat a little bit less, but eat in the same way you did before. That's a great way to start gaining all of the weight back.

Instead the best way to go about things is to continue eating in the same pattern that you were before. The only difference is that now you'll get to add in more calories.

So for example, if you were creating an average caloric deficit of 500 calories per day, then now you'll get to eat an additional 500 calories per day. If you were eating in a deficit of 300 calories per day, then this would mean that you could eat an extra 300 calories per day.

That's definitely something, but that can add up rather quickly. Maybe you can eat an extra serving of a side for lunch and dinner, or add in a couple of snacks.

If you want to think of it in another way, then take your resting metabolic rate and eat that many calories per day. In my case, this would mean that I would eat 2,691 calories per day.

The main point is that whatever it was you did to lose weight, you want to continue eating in that same pattern. Don't act as if anything is going to change.

And if you can't continue eating the way in which you lost weight, then your approach to weight loss probably wasn't that sustainable to begin with. The thing with the boiled egg diet is that you probably won't have to do the boiled egg diet once you reach your goal bodyweight.

You could continue to eat in the way you did when you were in the transition phase of the diet. The transition phase is what's going to be sustainable for you to do for a long time to come.

Conversely, the boiled egg diet is only something that you'll be able to do for short periods of time. If you ever find yourself in a situation where you need to lose a little bit of extra weight, then you can always turn back to the boiled egg diet as a quick solution.

However, once you do hit your target weight, you're much better off eating in a pattern similar to how you were eating during the transition phase, but simply adding in more calories.

Chapter 6: How to Incorporate Exercise with Your Diet Plan

The cool thing about losing weight is that you don't have to exercise if you don't want to. You can lose weight by focusing solely on your nutrition plan.

The boiled egg diet will work perfectly fine for you without you having to exercise. However, as you're going to see, there are some cool benefits that you can get from exercising that diet alone won't be able to provide you with.

Why Should You Exercise?

So if exercise isn't necessary for you to lose weight, then why should you do it? We're busy enough as it is, and exercising is one more thing to add to an already giant list of to-dos.

For starters, our bodies were designed for movement. Our ancestors were constantly on the move in order to find their next kill.

They were always on their feet walking, hunting, or gathering food. In the modern era, things are much different.

With advancements in technology, a lot of the work that people do now days is computer based. This means that more and more people are stuck sitting at a desk for eight hours a day.

You might not see the harm in this, but the research shows that people who are more sedentary are more likely to develop diabetes and heart disease among other things (3). Less and less people are working jobs where they're on their feet for most of the day, and this causes issues.

Exercising will help to correct some of these issues that we face from sitting in front of a computer for long hours at a time. Also like I just mentioned, exercise will help to reduce your risk for developing disease.

Yes getting down to a healthy body weight will also help to reduce your risk of disease, but why not maximize it with exercise. Being at a healthy body weight can only do so much for you.

Exercise will help to increase blood flow and circulation, which will help your body move blood cells and nutrients throughout your system easier. Not only that, but exercise will also help to give you a boost from a weight loss perspective.

Think about it—the main goal with weight loss is to create a caloric deficit. You can go about doing that in a couple of different ways—by exercising more and/or eating less.

You'll already have the eating less part down with the boiled egg diet. However, you can help to maximize your results by exercising.

Combining exercise with a diet plan will do one of two things for you—you'll either reach your goal faster, or you'll give yourself some extra leeway in your diet plan. For example, let's say that you're eating 1,700 calories per day in order to lose weight.

If you workout one day and burn 300 calories, then that means you could eat 2,000 calories for the day and still create the same caloric deficit. Or if you wanted, you could still eat the same 1,700 calories and create a deficit that's 300 calories larger than usual.

You can go about it whichever way you want to, but one thing is for certain—exercise will help you way more than it hurts you.

What Should You Do For Exercise?

If you do decide to exercise, then what should you do for exercise? There are many different options out there such as playing a sport, weight lifting, walking, cardio, etc.

One form isn't necessarily better than another; it really comes down to preference. At the end of the day, you have to do whatever you enjoy most because that's what you'll actually stick with.

With that being said, here are some different things that you can do for exercise:

Weight Lifting

Resistance training is my favorite form of activity. It's great for building strength and muscle.

It's also great for bone density as well, and lifting weights has been shown to help prevent and delay osteoporosis (4). Unfortunately, many people don't engage in lifting weights because they fear that it'll make them look like a bulky bodybuilder. You have to keep in mind though, that professional bodybuilders do what they do for a living, and most of them are enhanced with drugs.

It would be next to impossible to become as huge as most professional bodybuilders without enhancing drugs. If you're a natural lifter, engaging in resistance training will only improve the way your body looks, not hinder it.

In fact, if you want to build your best looking body possible, then you must lift weights. There's no other way around it.

Sometimes when people only use their diet to lose weight they aren't satisfied with how they look when they reach their goal bodyweight. This is because losing weight will help you get rid of any unwanted fat that you have, however it won't do anything to help you build muscle.

Muscle is what makes your body look firm and toned. If you only diet, then chances are that you'll end up looking flat and weak by the time you reach your goal.

On the other hand, if you combine diet with resistance training, then you'll look firm and fit when you hit your goal. Simply being skinny shouldn't be the goal if the reason why you want to lose weight is to look better.

If you want to look better and feel more attractive, then you need to incorporate some sort of resistance training into your routine as well. Lifting weights doesn't have to be complicated either.

As long as you focus on a few keys movements, you'll be good to go. Here's a weight routine you can follow if you're unsure of what to do in the weight room:

Workout Schedule:

This workout consists of 3 workouts per week. You'll perform the same workout each time you go to the gym.

Take at least one day of rest in-between workouts. Ideally you would workout on Monday, Wednesday, and Friday or Tuesday, Thursday, and Saturday.

Here's the actual workout:

- Dumbbell Forward Lunges 3 sets of 10 reps per leg (60 seconds rest between sets)
- Flat Dumbbell Bench Press 3 sets of 8 reps (90 seconds rest between sets)
- Wide Grip Lat Pulldown 3 sets of 8 reps (90 seconds rest between sets)
- Standing Dumbbell Military Press 3 sets of 10 reps (60 seconds rest between sets)
- Cable Tricep Kickback 3 sets of 12 reps (60 seconds rest between sets)
- Standing Dumbbell Curls 3 sets of 12 reps (60 seconds rest between sets)

There you have it! Don't be fooled by the simplicity of this workout! Regardless of your experience level you have with working out, this workout will be a challenge for you.

It all comes down to doing the best that you can and trying to lift more weight as time goes on. Not only that but if you are a complete beginner to lifting weights this workout is a great way to gain experience on some of the major lifts.

When you're new to resistance training, a lot of the battle is getting used to the form of the exercises. You might also be wondering what a set and a rep are.

A set is a group of consecutive repetitions. A repetition is one complete motion of an exercise.

And the rest period is how long of a break you'll take until you start the next set. For example, let's say you're completing sets of 10 reps and resting 60 seconds in between sets for the forward lunge exercise.

You'll lunge forward and stand back up, completing the movement of the exercise. Then you'll do the same for your other leg. This will complete one rep.

You'll repeat that motion 9 more times for a total of 10 repetitions. That will complete the set and you will begin your rest period. Once your 60-second rest period is up, you'll start the next set and perform another 10 repetitions.

That will complete set number 2, and you'll rest another 60 seconds. Once that time period is up, you'll complete the final set of 10 repetitions, and then you'll move onto the next exercise.

Usually, for most exercises, you won't have to complete reps for both sides of your body. For example, with the lat pulldown exercise, you'll pull the bar down towards your chest and then control the bar back up to the top position where your arms are fully extended. This will complete one rep.

Cardio

This is probably the most popular form of exercise for people who are interested in losing weight. This isn't necessarily a bad thing, but don't be fooled into thinking that just because it's popular for weight loss that means it's the most effective.

I find doing regular cardio on a treadmill to be boring so I avoid it most of the time. I'd rather do something else like playing basketball.

However, this doesn't mean that doing cardio on a treadmill won't be a good thing for you. Again it all comes down to doing what you enjoy the most because that's what will be easiest to stick with.

Cardio is great because it's a good way to burn some extra calories. Not only that, but it will also help to decrease your risk for cardiovascular disease and help to improve your conditioning if you're an athlete.

However, the one thing that cardio won't help you be able to do is build muscle. Even if you exercise and diet to reach your goal bodyweight, you still might not end up looking the way that you want to.

The reason for this is because cardio is great for burning fat, but it's not good for building muscle. Therefore, you're still going to end up looking flat when you reach your goal instead of firm and fit.

All in all, cardio is definitely worth doing if you want to burn some extra calories, but you need to go about doing it in the right way. Jogging for an endless amount of time isn't the most efficient way to go about things.

You can burn more fat in less time if you do high intensity interval training (HIIT for short) instead of long steady state cardio. Research has shown HIIT to be the most efficient form of cardio when it comes to fat loss (5)(6).

Essentially HIIT is a combination of going all out and going easy. For example, if you were to do a HIIT workout on a treadmill you might alternate between a speed of 8mph for 30 seconds and a speed of 3 mph for 1 minute.

And you would repeat that cycle for the duration of the workout, which would usually be around 10-20 minutes. And if you think about it, HIIT is essentially the exercise form of what we're doing with the boiled egg diet.

With the boiled egg diet there are periods of extreme weight loss followed by periods where you take it easy. This break gives your body the chance to catch up and prepare itself for the next boiled egg diet.

This is a similar pattern with HIIT. You have periods of intense exercise followed by periods of less intense exercise.

The less intense exercise periods allow your body time to rest and get ready for the next period of intense exercise. Of course, you're not bound to doing HIIT on a treadmill.

You can do HIIT on any cardio machine that you like such as an elliptical, stair master, rowing machine, or anything else you enjoy. You could even go outside and run if you like!

The main thing is that you alternate between a period of intense exercise and low intensity. Adjust time limits and speeds to match your current fitness level.

For example, if you're doing HIIT on a treadmill and 8 mph is too fast for you, then only run at 6 mph during your intense exercise periods. Or maybe you can run at 8 mph, but you can only keep it up for 15 seconds instead of 30 seconds.

That's totally fine! Run for 15 seconds instead of 30, and you can adjust the walk period as needed.

If you still need a minute of walking to recover then fine. If you only need 30 seconds, then take 30 seconds.

The key with the low-intensity part of the workout is to not take more rest than is necessary. The key with the high-intensity part of the workout is the push yourself as hard as you can for close to as long as you can. If you follow those guidelines when doing your HIIT cardio then you'll be good to go!

Playing Sports

This is my favorite way to do cardio. Any sport or game that you want to play that'll get your body moving will do the trick.

One isn't better than another. My favorite thing to do is play pickup basketball with my friends.

The cool thing about playing sports is that it's essentially HIIT cardio disguised in the form of a game. For example, in basketball, there are periods of intense running when you're trying to score a bucket or defend an opponent.

Then there are periods where you're taking a rest such as when the ball goes out of bounds and you're waiting for the inbounds pass. The same goes for soccer, tennis, and other sports that you may be interested in playing.

Walking

Walking is the last major category of exercise. Most fitness enthusiasts don't take walking very seriously, and I used to be one of these people.

I used to think that walking was only something that people who weren't in good shape did. I was so wrong about that!

Walking is great and everyone should be doing more of it. The first reason is that moving more will lower risk of developing cardiovascular disease (7).

Cardiovascular disease has never been higher, and one of the main reasons for it is because people are becoming more sedentary. Back in the day before the rise of corporations, people's jobs involved more movement and physical labor.

Now days, people aren't so lucky and are bound to a desk for eight hours a day. Even with that being the case, it's still important to find ways to walk more.

You could walk during your lunch break at work, start parking farther away when you go to stores, walk in the evening, or wherever else you can find the time. It doesn't have to be for a long time—even 10-15 minutes a day will do wonders for you!

Another great thing about walking is that it's the easiest form of exercise that you can do, and therefore it's the easiest way to burn additional calories. It doesn't involve changing your clothes and driving to the gym.

All you have to do is walk! Additionally walking is great for recovery and for your lymphatic system.

Your lymphatic system is responsible for detoxing your body, and it helps aid your body in recovery to different stresses among other things. The trick is, that your lymphatic system only works when you work.

You have to move in order to get your lymphatic system to move. That's why walking is great, and it's not for certain people—it's for everyone!

Chapter 7: Change the Way You View Dieting

When you break it down, all dieting comes down to is following a certain plan of action. Boom weight loss is that simple right?

Well no, not exactly. There's also a mental component that's involved with weight loss.

So far in this book, I've covered the mechanical things that you actually need to do in order to lose weight. This chapter is going to focus more on the psychological component of weight loss.

Don't neglect this because it could possibly be more important for you to get this right rather than the technical stuff.

What's Your Self-Image and Why It Matters

How do you view yourself? When you think of yourself do you usually think positive or negative things about yourself?

The reason why this matters is because your thought patterns could make or break your success. You see, you could have the best diet plan in the world, but if you don't view yourself as the type of person who's worthy or capable of losing weight, then you'll never achieve it.

Think about this. Your thoughts determine actions. Your actions determine your habits. And your habits will ultimately determine the kind of life that you live.

This can work for or against you depending on what your thoughts are. For example, if your general thought pattern is along the lines of not being worthy of achieving a fit body, then that will determine your actions.

You might not go to the gym because you don't think it'll benefit you at all. You eat a brownie because you're a lost cause etc.

These actions will then start to solidify into habits. You'll continue to take similar actions in the future.

Then once these habits are solidified, the feedback loop will repeat itself. Whenever you diet and something goes wrong (which it inevitably will) you'll tell yourself something like, "See I knew I wasn't cut out for this weight loss thing!"

The reality is that isn't the case, everyone experiences setbacks when they try to burn fat. The difference is that because you see yourself as someone who isn't capable of losing weight you only look for signs that validate your current beliefs.

You ignore anything that would show you really can achieve your goals. And the tough part about this is that a lot of it is subconscious, most of the time you're not even aware that you're sabotaging yourself.

Conversely you could view yourself as the type of person who is capable of achieving his or her goals. Sure you may have had a rough history with losing weight in the past, but your past doesn't have to determine your future unless you let it.

Thus, you decide that you will succeed. Making a firm decision is no joke.

To make a decision is to cut off any other possibilities. There is no other option.

With this type of determination, your actions will be much different from someone who views himself negatively. These positive actions will then determine your habits.

Your habits will determine your success. Then once something doesn't go your way, you'll be ready and you'll be able to bounce back and keep on going.

Therefore, your self image will make or break your success. You could have the drop-dead easiest diet plan in the world, but if your mindset isn't right, then it won't do you any good.

How to Improve Your Self-Image

Ok so now that you know your self-image may be an issue, what can you do in order to fix it? Well you've already taken a positive first step by reading the section above.

That's right, by being aware of your self-image you can start to change it. If you weren't aware of your self-image and the negative thoughts that you were feeding it, then it wouldn't be possible for you to change it.

The first step is awareness. You need to start becoming more aware of when these negative thoughts start to enter into your head.

Once you catch them, you can change them. What I like to do is when I notice a negative thought, I immediately think of a big red stop sign.

This way my mind will start to associate negative thoughts with a stop sign. You can think of anything you like that will help you stop the negative thoughts right in their tracks.

Then you'll want to replace that negative thought with a positive one. For example let's say you have this thought, "See I knew this diet wouldn't work for me!"

Once you have that thought, the first thing you need to do is become aware of it. Then picture a stop sign or something else that'll help get rid of that thought.

Finally, think of something positive. In this case, you could think of something like, "I did mess up my diet plan today, but I know I can bounce back and get even better results!"

Aside from that, here are some other things that you can do to help increase your self-image:

Give Yourself Permission to Be Human

Nobody's perfect. We all hear that and believe it to be true.

Yet when it comes to weight loss we act like everything has to be perfect. If I gained two tenths of a pound this week, then something must be wrong with me.

If I messed up and ate a slice of chocolate cake when I knew I shouldn't have, then I'll never let myself live it down. The thing is though we are all human, which means that we make mistakes! You have to embrace that!

Whatever goals you're trying to achieve, the path will not be smooth and easy. There will be bumps and potholes.

You'll end up going the wrong way at times. That's all ok and it will happen.

You have to have the right expectations going into a weight loss diet. Things aren't always going to be smooth, but if you know where you're going and are determined to get there, then nothing will stop you.

When you know that mistakes will happen, it's much easier to brush them off and keep on moving forward. Again the mistakes you've made in the past don't determine your future—remember that!

This is true even if you made a mistake five seconds ago! So let yourself be human and understand that it's ok to make mistakes from time to time.

You don't have to stay on track 100% of the time to get to where you want to go. Even if you're only able to follow the diet plan 85% of the time, that's way better than you think it is.

Believe it or not, airplanes only stay on course during 3% of the flight because the plane is zigzagging to the left and right of the straight path, and yet they almost always reach their end destination.

Following a diet 85% of the time will still be able to get you incredible results. And if you go into a diet expecting to be only 85% perfect, then things are going to be much easier when you do make a mistake.

Don't Compare Yourself to Others

This can be a hard thing to do, but it's definitely worth it. There's a biological urge in us to compare ourselves to others to see how we are stacking up.

We want to make sure that we fit in and that we won't fall too far behind. The thing is though that standards are completely made up.

Who says that you're a tall person if you're at least six feet tall? Who says you're rich if you have a million dollars?

These are standards that society has made up. What if you were only considered tall if you were seven feet tall? What if you were only considered to be wealthy if you had a net worth of a billion dollars?

Would anything actually be different? Of course nothing would be different except for the way you think about things.

You probably don't know of anyone who's a billionaire, but you might know of some people who are millionaires. If the standard was being a billionaire to be rich, you wouldn't feel bad about yourself because no one in your circle of friends is making that kind of money.

But instead the standard is a million dollars, and if someone you know has that kind of money, it'll make you feel like you're somehow a failure. This is why it's for the best to not compare yourself to others and focus on yourself and what it is that you need to do.

We all come from different backgrounds and different starting points. There could be a thousand reasons why someone is a millionaire and you aren't, so what?

Does someone else having more money than you change your life in the least bit? No of course it doesn't! Focus on yourself and the circumstances that you're currently dealing with.

Of course, going against this biological urge to compete and be the best can be a difficult thing to do. So how can we break it?

The first thing you need to do is cut back drastically on social media or ditch it altogether. The reason for this is that studies show that people who use social media more are more depressed than people who don't use social media (8).

The reason for this is because people are only posting the best things that are happening in their lives. Social media is a highlight reel of your friends' lives—Oh look I just got engaged!

Hey look at me I just got a sweet new job! Don't mind me, just hanging out with my perfect husband and 3 kids! Oh wow I just lost 20 pounds!

Meanwhile, you're on the other side wondering why you're still single, at a dead end job, and unable to lose weight. Do you really think seeing all of that is going to make you a happier and better person? No way!

And the sad thing is that most of it is exaggerated. If you only judged people by their social media postings, it would seem like everyone is happy.

Yet the research shows that millions of Americans struggle with depression (9). That's rather interesting isn't it?

Aside from that, the other thing you can do is focus more and more on your own goals. The more honed in you are on your own goals, the easier it is to mind your own business.

Most of the time when we divert our attention towards what's going on in other people's lives it's because we don't have much going on in our own lives. Live such an awesome life that you don't have time to think about what other people are doing.

I'm not saying that you should never know anything that's going on with your friends and that you should live under a rock for the rest of your life. What I am saying is that you need to be more choosy about the information you take in regarding other people in your life.

Why You Should Lose the Word Diet

The last thing you may want to consider doing to help improve your mindset is to drop the word diet from your vocabulary. Yes I know that I've been using the word diet throughout this book for the sake of simplicity, but there's a better way to think about it.

When you think of the word diet, what does that usually imply? It implies that you do something for a short period of time, then you stop doing it after awhile.

When you go on a diet, you must eventually come off of a diet. Of course, this doesn't necessarily have to be the case, but people go "on" diets all of the time and fail so it's hard to think of it differently.

Instead what you should think more about is lifestyle changes. If something is a part of your lifestyle then you're going to do it for the rest of your life.

Think of it like brushing your teeth. Brushing your teeth is something you do everyday without much thought behind it.

Your nutrition plan should be the same way. It should be something that you do as a part of your life.

It shouldn't be thought of as something temporary because you won't sustain any results that you achieve. That's why I want you to approach the boiled egg diet in the manner in which I've outlined it in the book.

This is the best way to make the boiled egg diet a lifestyle change and not a typical diet. If all you did was the two-week boiled egg diet, then you would only see short-term success and not long-term success.

The key to success with the boiled egg diet is what happens after the initial two weeks. If you're able to stay focused on the big picture, then you'll be much more likely to keep the weight off.

And if thinking of things in terms of a lifestyle change helps you out mentally, then by all means go for it. However, don't feel like you have to view things this way if you don't want to.

Chapter 8: Frequently Asked Questions

Can I Follow the Boiled Egg Diet Continuously?

You might think that it's a good idea to continue to follow the boiled egg diet week after week after week to get even faster results. However, this would be a mistake because you'd soon run your body into the ground.

Not only that, but you'd be fighting against some key fat-burning hormones in your body such as leptin. That's why it's best to follow the boiled egg diet in the manner that I've laid out in the book.

If you do the boiled egg diet and then follow it with a transition period, then your chances of losing weight and keeping it off will be much higher than if you only try to follow the boiled egg diet week after week.

Should I Focus More On Cardio or Weights if I Do Decide to Exercise?

You can do whatever you enjoy more because that's what will make you more likely to exercise in the first place. You can also do both weightlifting and cardio if you'd like.

The main thing here is to consider what you want to get out of the exercise. If you just want to burn some extra calories, get your heart rate up, and/or improve your conditioning, then cardio will get the job done.

On the other hand, if you want to firm up your muscles or even build muscle, then you'll want to lift weights. Lifting weights will still be a great way to burn calories and help aid in weight loss.

Do I Have to Exercise in Order to See Results with This Diet?

No, you certainly don't have to exercise in order to start seeing results with the boiled egg diet. I included a chapter on exercise so you'd have a plan for what you could do if you were interested, but it's not mandatory by any means.

You will be able to get results just from following the boiled diet by itself. Exercise will allow you to be able to get results faster or give you more leeway in your diet plan, which is pretty cool. So if you want to experience the benefits of exercise, then, by all means, do it.

What if I'm Not Losing Weight at 13 Calories per Pound of Bodyweight?

Let's say you calculate your resting metabolic rate by multiplying your bodyweight by 13. You still follow the boiled egg diet as it's laid out, but during the weeks when you're not following the boiled egg diet, your weight loss has stalled.

What should you do? The first thing to remember is that this really isn't that big of a deal.

Most of your weight loss should be occurring during the weeks when you're following the boiled egg diet. During weeks when you're not following the boiled egg diet, you're going to be eating in smaller caloric deficits or even at maintenance so weight loss won't be as great.

However, if you really want to, you can decrease your calories slightly more to help increase weight loss during the weeks when you're not doing the boiled egg diet. For example, you could start with 12 calories per pound of bodyweight, and then work your way down to 11 or even 10 calories per pound of bodyweight.

I know it can be tempting to want to cut your calories as low as possible, but once again, you need to remember the long game here. It's better to slow down and follow the boiled egg diet in a manner that'll allow you to be able to actually keep the weight off once you lose it.

I Gained Weight When I Started Eating More Calories. What Should I Do?

This is normal and should be expected, so the best thing you can do is not freak out and stay calm. The reason for this is because your bodyweight will fluctuate.

So when you're eating fewer calories, your glycogen stores will be lower. However, when you start to eat more calories, your muscles will fill up with more glycogen, which will cause a slight increase in bodyweight because glycogen isn't massless.

Therefore, you're not actually gaining fat here and that's why the number on the scale can be misleading. Don't be fooled by this and think that you always need to push yourself with eating low calories week after week because that'll only lead to burnout.

Instead be patient and realize that most of your weight loss will occur during the weeks when you're following the boiled egg diet. With that being the case, you may be tempted to do the boiled egg diet week after week, but remember we're seeking long-term sustainability here not quick results.

If you're going to be paranoid by the number on the scale, only weigh yourself once a week first thing in the morning after you use the bathroom. By weighing yourself in a consistent manner such as this, you'll be able to better judge if you've actually lost weight instead of just having to worry if your bodyweight is simply fluctuating.

Are There Any Supplements that I Should Take to Help Me Lose Weight?

The short answer to that is no, there are no supplements that you have to take in order to lose weight. Are there supplements out there that could give you a little boost? Yes.

Are they worth it? Probably not.

Companies that want your money have really overhyped supplements. They market their products to make it seem as if all you have to do is take this pill without doing anything else and boom you'll lose weight.

Deep down, we know it's not that easy, but we want it to be true so badly that we try it anyway. And that's why supplements companies make so much money.

They prey on people who aren't willing to do the hard (but necessary) stuff and who want the easy way out. I'm here to tell you that there is no easy way out.

You must follow sound nutrition and/or exercise principles in order to obtain your desired fitness result. I think you're better off skipping supplements and focusing on your diet plan as your main way of losing weight.

This isn't what supplement companies want you to hear, but it's the truth. Not only that, but think about what the word supplement means.

It's meant to supplement something (a sound diet or exercise plan in this case) not be a total replacement for it. Yet many people look to these supplements as magic, and they certainly are nothing of the sort.

With that being said, if you had some extra money on hand and there's a supplement you really want to try out, you certainly can. Just be cautious that you never buy a supplement with the expectations that it'll do all of the hard work for you because it certainly won't.

How Much Flexibility is There with the Boiled Egg Diet Meal Plan?

There's not too much flexibility with the boiled egg diet meal plan. There are reasons why you're eating the foods that you are.

Salads, fruits, vegetables, and eggs are very filling foods. They contain lots of vitamins, nutrients, and fiber, which will help to keep you fuller for a longer period of time.

So if you want to vary things a bit by eating vegetables instead of fruits or toast instead of a salad, then feel free to do so. For the most part however, stick to the plan as it's laid out.

Conclusion:

The boiled egg diet may not be the easiest thing you've ever done, but the results that you'll get are promising. The key is to stay focused on the long game.

Too many times people get caught up in short-term results and that causes them to fail in the end. Yes, the boiled egg diet will give you quick results to keep you motivated, but what you do when the boiled egg diet is over is the real key to your success.

Sources:

(1) https://www.ncbi.nlm.nih.gov/pubmed/13594881

(2) https://www.ncbi.nlm.nih.gov/pmc/articles/PMC4391809/

(3) https://www.ncbi.nlm.nih.gov/pmc/articles/PMC2857522/

(4) https://www.ncbi.nlm.nih.gov/pubmed/9927006

(5) http://www.ncbi.nlm.nih.gov/pubmed/18197184

(6) http://www.ncbi.nlm.nih.gov/pubmed/20473222

(7) https://www.ncbi.nlm.nih.gov/pmc/articles/PMC3098122/

(8) https://www.sciencedirect.com/science/article/pii/S0747563216307543

(9) https://www.nimh.nih.gov/health/statistics/major-depression.shtml